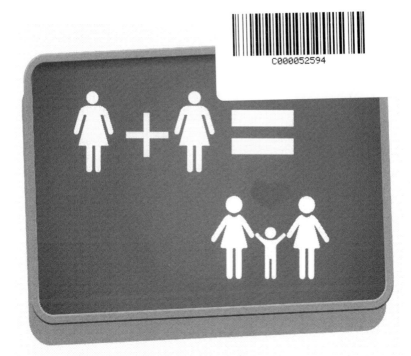

LESBIAN 101
CONCEPTION

An easy-to-follow, how-to get started guide for lesbians thinking about getting pregnant tomorrow or in a couple of years

KATHY BORKOSKI

Lesbian Conception 101

An easy-to-follow, how-to get started guide for lesbians thinking about getting pregnant tomorrow or in a couple of years

Kathy Borkoski

Lesbian Conception 101

An easy-to-follow, how-to get started guide for lesbians thinking about getting pregnant tomorrow or in a couple of years

© 2015 Kathy Borkoski

www.LesbianConception101.com

Dedicated to my wife, Lauren, and her willingness to go on this grand adventure of creating a family.

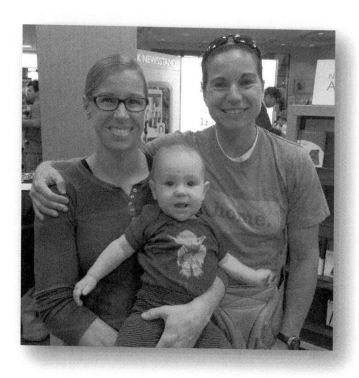

STOP! Before you go any further, don't forget to pick up your free gifts!

As a thank you for buying this book, I'd like to give you:

1. A Checklist for the Toughest Babymaking Decisions: Know where you stand so you can develop your plan!

Visit http://lesbianconception101.com/checklist

TABLE OF CONTENTS

Chapter 1. We Want to Have a Baby... Now What?

Thank you for purchasing this book! I'm excited to share with you everything Lauren and I learned on our journey to start a family. When we first decided it was time to put our plan for a family into action, I was floored at **how much information there was out there** - and I felt like I was missing the magic decoder ring to understand what all the websites were trying to tell me.

It took us a year of trying, eight inseminations, countless ovulation tests, and a lot of chlomid-induced mood swings before we finally got pregnant. In that time, I learned a TON about the many different techniques and costs associated with trying to get pregnant.

I googled, read books, researched infertility treatments, and asked doctors, friends, and random women that I met in the gym question after question until I had a pretty good idea of how everything worked. (You will be shocked how many of your straight friends have had fertility issues... and they know you're not doing it the "natural" way so they'll tell you all about it!) During that time, we definitely made costly mistakes and missed out on opportunities that may have sped up the process.

Once we became pregnant, I started getting a lot of questions from friends about all the details and decisions we made. I recommended books they could read, but **my friends just wanted someone to break**

everything down into the basics so they knew where to start researching.

So I wrote this simple guide that breaks down the basics and gives lesbians like me and my wife a place from which to start making decisions.

I keep it simple and straightforward. I include all those (seriously!) awkward questions your straight friends will ask you. And most importantly, it's short enough that you'll read it but give you enough information to feel confident about getting started.

This is not an end-all-be-all guide to insemination, nor is it a doctor approved, guaranteed-to-get-pregnant, hard-to-understand-without-a-medical-degree book. It is designed to be a guide to get you started on the right foot for your situation and give you a lot of things to think about (that I wish we'd known in advance!).

Whatever method(s) you decide on, it only needs to be the right choice for your family. Everyone around you will have an opinion and offer their recommendations, but do your best to focus inward on you and your partner and determine what is best for the two of you!

Note: This information is only a guide to the basics, lingo, and costs. Check with your doctor, cryobank, fertility center, specific product directions, and other medical resources for specifics.

Real Stories: What do you wish you'd known when you first got started?

Pregnancy is hard. It is never guaranteed and it's VERY emotional. The ups and downs, hopes and disappointment with every "try" can be taxing personally and on the relationship. So try to be gentle and PATIENT with yourself and your partner. Also, no matter how much reading you do, or how much you think you know your cycle and body, you are likely off in some very significant ways. Lastly, enjoy it as much as possible! All of it. You likely won't remember most of it two years later (like us). – Kayla and Lisa

I knew this but want to make sure others do- don't waste your time with at home inseminating with frozen sperm. I don't know anyone who has actually gotten pregnant that way. Waste of time and money! – Tara and Tanya

I wish we'd known the emotional toll of failed attempts. – Asha and Marissa

Dispelling Preconceived Notions

I had a lot of preconceived notions when it came to making a baby that I'm very happy to tell you aren't necessarily true. The horror stories you hear in the news about huge expenses and legal battles with sperm donors don't have to be true for you if you take appropriate precautions. Here's a list of some of the things I thought were true (don't worry, I cover why all of these aren't true later in the book!):

Fallacy 1: *Making a baby is insanely expensive.* I knew there were different kinds of insemination but I assumed all of them would cost me tens of thousands of dollars. We had been saving in case things really were that expensive but were really excited when we found the method that was right for us and allowed us to make our baby for less than $3,000.

Fallacy 2: *I can't use a known donor because of all the legal issues.* It turns out, there are a lot of ways to protect yourself if you decide to go this route. Additionally, there are many more reasons to go with an unknown donor than just the legal concerns than we originally realized (I mean, it's just sperm, right?!).

Fallacy 3: *No one will understand what we're going through.* I was shocked at how many straight friends, even really close ones, I had that told us their infertility stories when we announced we were trying to have a baby. It turned out that even when you have all the right organs in a relationship, there are still problems and stresses.

Fallacy 4: *I have no history of infertility, so it should work on the first or second time.* When it took me a year of trying, I began to think there was something wrong with me despite the doctor's assurances to the contrary. When I read up on pregnancy stats, I was surprised to find out that even in the best of circumstances the success rate is somewhere around 10-20%.

How to Use this Book

I know you're tempted to read every word of this book as though it were the latest Harry Potter (or at least I would be very flattered if you did!), but instead, think of it as a workbook. At the end of each chapter, I give you assignments which include conversations to have with each other and things to research.

By the end of this book, hopefully you have a good idea of the way you want to make a baby along with some good ideas on how to take better care of yourself, get on the same page as your partner/wife, and avoid unnecessary expenses.

Chapter 1 Assignment: Sit down with your future co-parent and talk about the things you worry about for having a baby. Get it all out in the open. And then talk about all the reasons you're excited to have a baby with her and start reading this book to figure out how you're going to do it.

Note: Wine and romance is always recommended for this type of conversation. Enjoy each other before you make your new roommate(s)!

Chapter 2. Lesbian Babymaking Dictionary: New Words that Describe your Reproductive Parts, Cycle, and the Process

You and your partner decide it is time to have a baby. You meet with your regular doctor, are referred to a fertility clinic to discuss your options, and after your first appointment you are left in a state of bewilderment, and possibly even a "*you are going to do what to my what now?*" feeling. Understanding the language involved in the conception process can be quite confusing, so here are some of the basic terms you are likely to encounter but may not completely understand the importance of, even if you've heard the terms before.

Artificial Insemination: The general term for the procedure in which sperm is inserted into a woman's cervix or uterus. This includes IntraCervical Insemination (ICI), IntraUterine Insemination (IUI), and In Vitro Fertilization (IVF) and is the whole reason you picked up this book.

Basal Body Temperature (BBT): The body temperature of a person immediately upon awakening, before any activity used to help chart a woman's ovulation.

Cycle: The time frame from the first day of one period to the next. This cycle includes the maturation of the egg, release of the egg, and the thickening of the uterine lining in preparation for a fertilized egg. If fertilization or conception does not occur then menstruation begins, the lining and egg are removed from the body, and the cycle begins again.

Cervical Mucus: Mucus produced by the cervix that increases as ovulation approaches. You will get very familiar with your mucus during this process.

Cervix: The lower section and opening of the uterus that protrudes into the vagina - the gateway to the uterus.

Clomid: A drug that can stimulate the ovaries to produce more/larger eggs.

Cryobank/spermbank: A facility that can store frozen sperm and eggs. Many also have banks of sperm donors.

Cryotank: A cooler, typically filled with liquid nitrogen that can keep sperm frozen for up to 7 days.

Follicle: A group of cells forming a cavity in the ovary where an egg will form. When you get an ultrasound, your doctor may reference "chocolate chip cookie." This is because the follicles in the ovary are dark spots on your ovary and it kind of looks like a chocolate chip cookie.

IntraCervical Insemination (ICI): An artificial insemination technique in which sperm are put onto a woman's cervix.

IntraUterine Insemination (IUI): An artificial insemination technique in which sperm are put directly into a woman's uterus.

In Vitro Fertilization (IVF): An assisted reproductive technique that involves removing sperm and eggs, fertilizing them in a laboratory, then placing a fertilized egg in the uterus.

Luteinizing Hormone: A hormone that triggers ovulation.

Ovulation: One stage in your cycle – the stage in which an egg can be fertilized.

Leutenizing Hormone (LH) Surge: A spontaneous release of large amounts of LH during a woman's menstrual cycle. This normally results in the release of a mature egg from a follicle (ovulation). May also be referred to as the "surge."

Vaginal Ultrasound: The use of high-frequency sound to create images of your insides. For fertility treatments, sonograms are typically done vaginally (think magic wand that inserts into your vagina).

Vial: A small, sealed tube with one dose of sperm.

Chapter 2 Assignment: Practice saying all these words out loud with a straight face.

Chapter 3. The First Steps

Before you can execute any of the information in this book, it will be helpful if you get a clear picture of where you currently stand today. This clear picture will push you in the direction of certain options and away from others.

Step 1: Call your insurance company and learn about what is and is not covered. Our insurance provider covered all the expenses of a baby, but none of the fertility treatments. However, they did cover certain drugs I was prescribed over the course of our fertility treatments.

Step 2: Analyze your budget. Do you need to start saving more before you can get started? Later chapters will go into the exact costs of the different types of babymaking options. Understanding where you stand financially will help you figure out which methods are best for you.

Step 3: Google and call fertility clinics in your area and start creating a cost spreadsheet for their services.

Step 4: Read the rest of this book and then start making some decisions!

Chapter 3 Assignment: Start working on steps 1, 2, and 3.

Real Stories: How did you start learning about how to get pregnant?

We did a lot of reading and went through a lot of trial and error! – Kayla and Lisa

We read several books and we asked around about the best fertility clinic in our area. – Tara and Tanya

We visited a fertility doctor to verify my fertility and have a backup plan. – Asha and Marissa

Chapter 4. Sperm: The Missing Ingredient

For lesbian couples, there is a key factor missing in the fertilization equation: sperm.

So aside from understanding your own body, there are some sperm handling procedures, terminology, and facilities you'll encounter in the hunt for donor sperm.

What Cryobanks Do With Sperm

Cryobanks collect and store sperm from donors for use in artificial insemination. If you are looking for an unknown donor, most of them have websites you can look through to find your perfect donor. If you have a known donor, you can have them donate to the cryobank for you to ensure the sperm is checked for communicable diseases and washed for the type of insemination you will use. Also, using the cryobank as an intermediary between you and the donor can provide additional legal protections depending on your state of residence.

After a donation, the ejaculate is checked for communicable diseases and motility, "washed," and split into vials based on sperm count and motility/progression. Many cryobanks aim to have 10 million sperm cells per vial and the amount of sperm in each man's ejaculate can vary greatly. This means one donation can be 1 vial or 10 vials. The average number of vials per ejaculate is around 4-5 depending on the prep type. The term "washed" means that the sperm is separated from the mucus and non-motile sperm in the semen to improve the chances of fertilization and to extract certain disease-carrying material in the semen.

Cost Saving Tip: Check with your cryobank to find out if they have discounts around the number of vials you purchase and free storage.

Once split up, the sperm is frozen in small vials (smaller than your thumb) using liquid nitrogen. The cryobank stores the vials until you are ready for insemination. If you are using a known donor, you will pay for storage from the beginning. If you are using an unknown donor, you will pay for storage from the day you purchase the sperm.

Many couples purchase several vials of sperm for use throughout the months and multiple tries it will take them to get pregnant. When purchasing sperm, the cryobank may offer different deals around numbers purchased and a year of free storage. Purchasing an extra vial to reach the number for free storage could save you hundreds more in the first year of free storage. If you don't end up using all the vials, you can usually sell back the unused ones.

One reason to not take the free storage option would be if the cryobank is far from your house and requires shipping. Shipping a cryotank can cost around $200 and be tricky to time for ovulation due to the 1-3 day lead time needed. A local cryobank would be much easier and more flexible for pickups. Cryotanks are usually good for around 7 days, so if you decide to stay with the distant cryobank and do the shipping option, you can arrange shipment a couple days prior to expected ovulation.

How to Work with Cryobanks When You're Inseminating

Knowing how cryobanks work can also help alleviate some stress on the day of insemination.

The vials of sperm are stored in cryotanks, and the cryotanks are generally checked out when you request the sperm. The tank keeps it frozen during transport, or is used to store the sperm at home if you predict you will be ovulating when cryobanks may not be open. Cryotanks are surprisingly large (1-3 feet tall) and need to be kept upright so the liquid nitrogen doesn't spill. I was insanely paranoid about the tank tipping over so I would buckle it in when I drove!

If you have a general idea of when you will ovulate, you can call your cryobank a week or so in advance to have them set aside a tank for you when you expect to pick up the sperm in case they are close to running out. If you think you'll ovulate over the weekend, pick the sperm up by Friday. Though a doctor should be consulted first, some people have stored sperm in coolers with dry ice just prior to their insemination appointment when no cryotanks are available.

Chapter 4 Assignment: Research donor sites and cryobanks to find the most cost-effective solution for your situation.

Real Stories: Sperm Decisions

If you think there is a possibility you will have more than one child, buy and preserve extra sperm. We didn't and our donor is no longer available so our son would have a different donor than his sibling if we ever decide to have another. – Tara and Tanya

Chapter 5.   Picking the Donor that is Right for You

We all wish that we could combine our genes with those of our partner/wife, and maybe that will be possible in a couple years or decades, but not now. So as lesbians, we have to choose the other half of our baby's gene pool. Whether you select a known or unknown donor, there are many things to consider.

Family medical history

For unknown donor sperm, family medical history is handled by the cryobank. For a known donor, you will need to do your own due diligence. Genes are responsible for not only the way we look, but also everything else about us, both good – intelligence, athletic ability, and healthiness, and bad – biological disorders, cognitive and developmental impairments, and health conditions. A thorough family medical history will identify health conditions in the donor and their close family (parents, grandparents, and siblings) that exceed the normal population. Family medical history can help identify patterns in families that may be red flags and indicate that there is an increased the likelihood that a health condition is hereditary.

Appearance

Hair color, eye color, skin color, ethnicity, height, weight, personality traits, and body type are all traits that can be easily identified as part of genetic gift we get from our parents. If you are on the hunt for a good donor, a major consideration may be what the donor looks like because you want your child to look similar to both you and your partner. Of course, there is no guarantee on which parent's genes will express more loudly (which is why some kids look like mom, some look like dad, and some don't really look like either). But you can plan to at least try to match key aspects of your partner to those of your donor.

Background

Is a college degree important to you in a donor? Or athleticism, musical ability, or creativity? There's a broad range of things people have in their life history that we would love to see in our children. For an unknown donor, there are cryobanks that collect this information and give you the ability to search by it.

Quantity of sperm donations

It's hard to know how many vials of sperm you will need. You could get pregnant on the first try or after 14 tries. Additionally, after you get pregnant, you may want to have enough on hand for when you are ready to have your second child. Many couples each want to get pregnant, but they'd like to do so using the same donor so that the children would genetically be half-siblings. How many vials the cryobank has on hand for a certain donor becomes very important in these situations. Additionally, many will tell you if a certain donor would be open to donating more in the case that the bank ran out.

Considerations for purchasing more sperm than you think you are going to need typically revolve around cost. Purchasing more sperm in the beginning means more upfront payment for a larger number of vials. If you are going to hold vials of sperm for a second pregnancy, you will need to pay for the storage time between pregnancies.

Type of Sperm (Prepared for ICI or IUI)

Depending on the type of artificial insemination you select (covered in detail in a later chapter), the sperm will need to be prepared to certain levels. Sperm prepared for IUI has been through an extra "wash" and can be used for ICI or IUI. Sperm prepared for ICI will need to go through some additional procedures to be ready for IUI. Your fertility center will be able to do the extra washing procedures required to take the sperm from ICI- to IUI-ready, but there may be an extra expense associated with it.

Open or Closed Unknown Donor

Some cryobanks have worked with their donors to determine if they would be willing to meet their genetic offspring at a much later date. This does not mean that they be involved in any way with raising the child, but rather that if requested by the adult offspring, the donor would allow for a meeting. This is known as an Open Donor. A Closed Donor has indicated that he would not be open to ever meeting the offspring resulting from his sperm donation.

Known vs Unknown Donor

In addition to all the attributes of a donor above, one of the largest decisions around donated sperm is whether or not you know the donor. Many couples want to be 100% certain that there is no other person that could claim any parental rights. Or some couples want there to be a genetic family connection to both partners. Below are some of the major advantages to each.

Advantages to an Unknown Donor:

- Much stronger legal protections
- More genetic testing and family history costs shouldered by the cryobank
- Potentially greater comfort for the non-carrying partner
- Can be more selective of specific attributes without offending anyone
- No awkward family interactions if the donor was a partner's brother
- No concerns around an outside person believing their opinion matters to the way you choose to raise your child
- Some cryobanks will have pictures of the donor when they were a child, but few have pictures of them as an adult

Advantages to a Known Donor:

- If you do want the child to know where their genes came from
- If you believe the child would be advantaged by some degree of relationship with their genetic contributant

- If a health issue were to arise with the child, the donor can be contacted to determine if it is in the genetic family history
- Can see what traits the child received from the donor
- Would be able to introduce the child to the donor if they asked for it
- Can learn a great deal more about the donor, including personality, lifestyle, and interests
- You will know what the donor looks like as an adult

Chapter 5 Assignment: Go through each of the sections in this chapter together and discuss what aspects are important to you. You may want to prioritize criteria together now so that when good candidates are found, you'll more easily be able to select the one that is best for your family.

Real Stories: How did you pick a donor?

Our donor choice was comprised of many factors. But most importantly, health and education history. We also wanted height. Our families are not traditionally tall or lengthy and we wanted to do our best to "stretch" those possibilities out. As for features, we chose mine because I was planning on carrying Lisa's egg (if I was carrying my own egg, we would have gone with Lisa's features). So, we chose features similar to mine, plus one foot of height. – Kayla and Lisa

We selected a cryobank and then looked for profiles that matched Tanya's physical description. Our goal was to create a child that would look like he came from both of

us. After we found several profiles we loved, we brought them home at Christmas time and had our families vote on the ones they liked. We found our winner that way!
  – Tara and Tanya

We had 2. The first was a friend of a friend that had a great spirit and needed some money; several attempts were unsuccessful. Our second donor is a wonderful friend who is like a brother to me and wanted to bless us. He is gay as well. – Asha and Marissa

Chapter 6. Deciding Who Should Carry

Some couples just know the answer to this question. And others agonize over it. Here are some of the criteria other couples have used to figure out who will carry first, second, or at all:

- **Age**. Especially in the case where one partner is older.
- **Desire to carry**. In some couples, one partner is dying to carry and one has little to no interest. And with IVF, even the partner that doesn't want to carry can still be the egg donor.
- **Health issues**. Our health can dictate how prepared our body is to get pregnant. One partner may be experiencing a health issue that will make it challenging or impossible to get pregnant at a certain time, but the couple still wants to start a family.
- **Genetic disorders**. Some partners have a genetic disorder or trait they don't want to pass on to their child.
- **Job or life situation**. We can't make our own baby independently, but we do have the option of two wombs in our relationships! Sometimes the positions each of us are in at specific stages of life/career make it easier or more difficult to be pregnant or focus on a baby.
- **Fertility issues**. Sometimes we just don't know why some women can get pregnant on the first

try and others can't get pregnant or miscarry. As a lesbian couple, our advantage is that we have a second womb to try for success with!

Chapter 6 Assignment: Make a plan for who is going to try to get pregnant and in what order.

Real Stories: How did you decide who would carry?

At the time, my job was more flexible and my insurance plan was better. We weren't sure when Lisa's job would be more stable or predictable and we weren't getting any younger, so we decided that I would carry. – Kayla and Lisa

I always joke (but it's actually not joking) that we would have ended up divorced before the baby was even born if Tanya carried. Tanya is a bit of a hypochondriac and has some back issues to boot. Plus, I really wanted to carry!! – Tara and Tanya

My biological clock was kicking and screaming. And Lauren was more than happy to let me carry first. Lauren still isn't thrilled with the idea of carrying now that we've had one, so we think I'll probably carry the next time, too, but with Lauren's egg. – Kathy and Lauren

My wife carried because I delivered children in a previous relationship. – Asha and Marissa

---

Chapter 7. Upping Your Chances of Success – Tracking Your Cycle

Contrary to what we are taught in high school Sex Education and on MTV's 16 and Pregnant, for many women, getting pregnant is not as easy as it seems. Unlike men, women are only fertile a few days out of each month or cycle. For lesbian couples, there is no accidental pregnancy (no matter how hard you try!). To succeed with artificial insemination, everything must be timed according to a fertility cycle. Not timing a cycle right can not only lead to an unachieved pregnancy but can also be very costly and emotionally frustrating. In addition to selecting the artificial insemination method that is best for you, it is helpful to have a healthy dose of humor and patience, along with some ground knowledge of the female fertility cycle.

The Ovulation Cycle

In general, a woman's monthly cycle is around 28 days long. However, some women will experience longer cycles, such as 40 days, and some may have shorter cycles closer to 21 days. Every woman is different and even the time for an individual woman's cycle can vary from one cycle to the next depending on many factors, including stress (like the stress of trying to get pregnant and manage expenses!). Ovulation is when an egg is released from its follicle in the ovary and travels through the fallopian tubes. The time period in which ovulation occurs in a woman's cycle varies, but it tends to be twelve to sixteen days prior to the next period, and you only have about a 12 to 24 hour window in which the egg can be fertilized.

Cycle day one, often abbreviated as CD1 in charting software, marks the first day of the menstrual period. Although many books and doctors will tell women to time insemination at about CD14, this haphazard guessing of when ovulation will occur is often not specific enough when dealing with frozen sperm and expensive doctor visits and can lead to unnecessary failure. As some women can ovulate as early as CD7 or even as late as CD28, it is important that women learn about their bodies and cycles to achieve a pregnancy in a more timely and less frustrating fashion.

Real Stories: Ovulation

I thought tracking ovulation would be easy – pee on a stick, tell the doctor it was positive. But for me, my cycle has always varied from 22 – 25 days and I wasn't getting a positive when we expected. So my doctor had me test in the morning and night starting at day 10 for a cycle. This helped us figure out where in my cycle it happens and I was finally able to consistently get a positive reading for future cycles by testing every morning when we got close. – Kathy and Lauren

For the first time ever, we realized that ovulation is NOT simple, nor guaranteed! I personally ovulated late in my cycle (around day 20 of 30, or 18 of 28), which we also learned effects progesterone levels. Needless to say, I had to take the maximum allowable shot of progesterone before and during the first 14 weeks of my pregnancy to assure the baby would stick. – Kayla and Lisa

Your Cycle's First Half

During the first part of a woman's cycle, the body is preparing an egg to be fertilized. Under the influence of several different pituitary hormones, including estrogen, follicles develop in the ovaries. They grow bigger and as the cycle continues, usually only one becomes dominant. It is this one that will release an egg at the time of ovulation and the others will recede and be absorbed back into the ovaries. If you have an ultrasound during this phase, your doctor may use the term "chocolate chip cookies." This is because your ovaries look like light circles on the ultrasound screen and the follicles with potential eggs are dark spots on the light circles.

The growing follicle produces the estrogen hormone, which signals the body to produce luteinizing hormone (LH). When enough estrogen has been produced, an LH surge occurs causing the mature egg to be released in 12-36 hours. This egg release is otherwise known as ovulation.

If you read the fertility websites for straight couples, you'll read that the most fertile time period during a woman's cycle is a few days before ovulation and a day or two after. This is because fresh sperm can survive for as long as five days in the female reproductive tract, awaiting the release of the egg, and also because the egg will live about 12-36 hours after it has been released. The key thing to note is that this is for fresh sperm. Studies have been done on frozen sperm showing that they typically only survive 12-24 hours in the female reproductive tract. So for lesbians, the type of donor sperm selected plays a role in how important it is to get the timing as right as possible. If you are doing doctor assisted ICI or IUI with frozen sperm, you will be told to track your body very closely for your LH surge. When the surge occurs, you call the doctor and make the insemination appointment for the next day.

Rough time estimates:

- LH Surge: 12-36 hours before egg is released (ovulation)
- How long the egg is viable: 12-24 hours
- How long thawed sperm survives in the uterus: 12-24 hours
- How long fresh sperm survives in the uterus: up to 72 hours

Signs that Ovulation is Approaching

As the female body prepares for ovulation, many changes occur due to an increase in estrogen. The cervix becomes softer and opens in preparation for any sperm that might come calling. Cervical fluid becomes greater in quantity and wetter. Closer to ovulation cervical fluid changes to an egg-white type consistency, which will help aid sperm through the hostile environment to the awaiting egg. To be better prepared and know when an artificial insemination should be done, women can track their cervical mucus and cervical texture. The more experience they have doing this, the better the chances of getting pregnant are, as timing will be more accurate.

Another tool for tracking fertility are ovulation test kits or testing strips. Ovulation test kits look a lot like home pregnancy tests and test strips look like the test strips you used in chemistry class. The test kits are just a much fancier version of the test strips, giving you an easier to understand readout. If you read the packaging, both methods are easy to use and test strips are about 1/20th the cost of the full test kit (which becomes really important when you have to test many times each cycle). Both methods test your urine for the presence of LH. When an LH surge has occurred and the test is positive, an insemination should be done within the time periods mentioned previously. Doctors can also perform blood tests to determine when an LH surge is occurring though home tests are usually quite accurate, less expensive, and more convenient.

If you've been peeing on the sticks or strips and not having much luck getting an indication that you are surging, try testing before you go to sleep and first thing when you wake up. When you first wake up, your pee is more concentrated, so even if there are lower amounts of LH, you should get an indication. For me, I hadn't had success identifying my LH surge with the test strips for the first two inseminations. So I spent the next cycle (per my doctor's recommendation) testing a lot until I got an indication on the test strips. I started testing early (around CD10) both before I went to bed and when I got up. I got my first LH surge indication on a test strip on the evening of CD13. From then on, I didn't have any issues tracking my LH surge with the test strips and I made sure I was using the cheapest testing option!

Another method of tracking ovulation is by keeping a chart of your basal body temperature (BBT). A basal body temperature is the temperature of the body at rest. This should be done first thing upon waking in the morning, prior to getting out of bed. Getting up to use the restroom, taking a drink, or other small activities can cause this method to not be accurate. Prior to ovulation, the temperature will be lower. Immediately after ovulation, the basal body temperature will increase, usually by at least 0.3 to 0.5 of a degree and will remain higher until the luteal phase is over, or through the duration of the pregnancy, if one has occurred.

BBT will not indicate that ovulation is approaching though some women will notice a slight dip in their BBT the day of or before ovulation. However, it is a strong indicator that ovulation has occurred. Women wishing to incorporate this method into getting pregnant will need to be committed to doing so. The BBTs of several weeks, or even months, must be looked at as a big picture, as individual days alone will not give an indication of when ovulation has occurred or will occur. Looking at a pattern over time will help most women get a clear picture of when they are most likely to ovulate in their cycle. I've heard of many women successfully using BBT to track ovulation; however, I was not one of those women. No matter how hard I tried, I always remembered to take my temperature after I'd already gotten up to pee!

The Luteal Phase

The second half of the fertility cycle, also known as the luteal phase, is ruled by progesterone, thanks to the follicle that released the egg. Whether conception has occurred or not, progesterone will cause any cervical fluid to quickly dry up after ovulation, the basal body temperature to remain higher, and the cervix to close and become firm again. It will also prevent menstruation from occurring. If conception has occurred, progesterone will increase and help maintain the pregnancy. If a pregnancy has not been achieved, the follicle will decrease in size and be reabsorbed by the body, causing a drop in progesterone. This drop will signal that body that it is time for a new cycle to begin and the woman's period will start. The luteal phase lasts between 9-14 days though a luteal phase less than 12 can be a sign of fertility issues that can impact the likelihood of pregnancy.

Charting the LH surge, BBT, cervical fluid, and cervical texture and position throughout the entire ovulation cycle can help know when an artificial insemination should be done. It can be very empowering for women to know more about their bodies and know that there are steps they can take to improve their chances of a pregnancy, and in turn decrease stress and the amount of money spent on getting pregnant.

Bottom Line: Learning as much as you can about your body and when you are most likely to ovulate will improve your timing and potentially reduce the number of tries (and the amount of money) for you to get pregnant.

Chapter 7 Assignment: Grab some ovulation kits and start tracking your cycle for a couple of months before you are ready to start inseminating!

Chapter 8. ICI, IUI, IVF... WTF? The Major Types of Artificial Insemination

There are a lot of choices out there and if you haven't thought about how babies are made since Sex Education class it can get a little confusing. But not to fear, I'm going to break down the basics for each type of insemination and give you some things to consider when selecting the form best for you.

The options range on a scale from at home, cheap procedures with a known donor, to expensive fertility treatments with anonymous sperm donors at a doctor's clinic. The most popular options are ICI, IUI or IVF. Each treatment has its benefits and downsides and it ultimately depends on your circumstances.

Now, grab a pen and paper to take notes and let's get started!

IntraCervical Insemination (ICI)

This type of insemination is the closest to the old turkey baster joke. I think there's a good chance a man came up with this joke – because, seriously, have you seen the size of a turkey baster? Who else but a man would think they could fill that thing!

Description: The most affordable and simplest option. This method is closest to the natural way (a penis) of delivering sperm to the uterus, only using different equipment, generally a syringe. The sperm is deposited into the cervical canal and proceeds to navigate the cervix, uterus, and end in the fallopian tubes naturally.

Type of Sperm: For this procedure, sperm can be used as is (fresh) or it can be washed. When it is washed, it removes harmful chemicals known as prostaglandins (think of these as potential STD carriers), as well as any sperm that is less likely to survive through the cervix.

Note: If the sperm donor you chose only has IUI vials available, these can also be used for ICI treatments as this just means the sperm was washed an extra time.

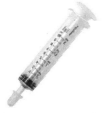

At home process: When you receive the sperm in the liquid nitrogen cryotank, carefully remove the vial per the instructions making sure to use an oven mit or other protector for your skin when handling the metal pieces. Next, take the vial and warm it up to room temperature in your hand. Once all the sperm is thawed, or if you are using fresh sperm, use the needleless, plunger-type syringe to draw up the sperm. Point the tip up towards the ceiling and tap the syringe to get the air bubbles to the top, then push the plunger in until all the air bubbles are out. Get into a comfortable position you can stay in for 10 or 15 minutes. Then you can 1) insert the syringe into the vagina and up close to the cervix without trying to go into it, or 2) use a speculum to see the cervix and position the syringe close to the opening of the cervix.

Finally, you will gently squeeze the sperm out of the syringe and onto or close to the cervix.

At the doctor: The same general process is followed at the doctor but they will handle all the sperm preparation and insemination. Additionally, the doctor will use a speculum and make sure the sperm is deposited into an optimal position. Typically, the doctor will also help your partner make the actual insemination with the syringe if you so desire.

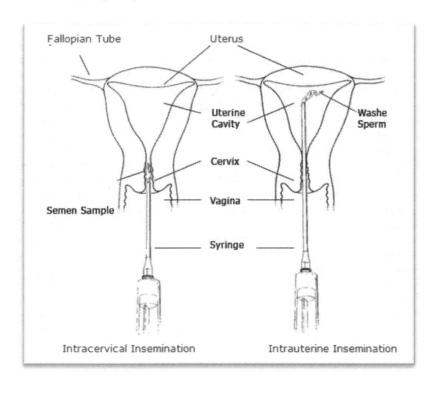

Image Source:
http://www.fertilityindia.com/husband_insemination.php

Reasons for Choosing ICI: This is a great option for lesbian couples that have no known fertility issues as they do not need the assistance of hormones or medical professionals. And it has the potential to have the least impact on your budget. However, it also provides the least insight and guidance into what your body is doing which may result in more tries to get the timing right (more tries = more sperm = more expense).

Real Stories: ICI

We naturally conceived twins via "turkey baster" courtesy of a wonderful donor. We literally used an infant medicine dispensing syringe. – Asha and Marissa

For our first 4 attempts, we did at-home ICI. We were very lucky to have neighbors who happened to be lesbian doctors with a 6-month son (talk about amazing neighbors!) who talked us through the entire process and made us feel confident about trying it at home. The procedure was much easier than we expected. The only thing I would have done differently in retrospect is had all 5 vials we purchased from the California Cryobank shipped to a local cryobank storage facility. For each insemination, we had them FedEx 1 vial to us. At $180 per shipment ($220 if we needed it the next day), the additional cost quickly added up. – Kathy and Lauren

---

IntraUterine Insemination (IUI)

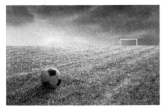 I think of this fertility type as playing soccer without a goalie because the sperm is deposited past the cervix and

33

directly into the uterus. If you're curious about how the cervix is like a goalie, google cervical mucus and position to learn more about the role the cervix plays in your fertility.

Description: IUI, or IntraUterine Insemination, goes one step further than ICI by depositing the sperm directly into the uterus rather than into the cervix. The cervix has natural defenses designed to actually prohibit sperm entering the uterus until the timing is right. And for some women, a hostile cervix can be a barrier to pregnancy.

While the sperm still have to navigate the rest of way, they are at least in a better position for achieving fertilization. Additionally, bypassing the cervix will allow more sperm to reach their destination, leading to a higher chance of fertilization because the cervix filters out slower or weaker sperm, so less make it to the final destination.

Type of Sperm: For IUI procedures, the sperm has to be washed to remove the seminal fluid (unwashed sperm placed in the uterus can cause the inseminated woman harm). This may happen at the cryobank that stores the sperm, or the clinic may thaw and wash the sperm prior to an insemination appointment. This is part of what makes IUI more expensive than ICI treatments: the sperm must be washed an extra time and the procedure must be performed by a doctor.

Basic Process: This process can involve multiple appointments because with IUI, the timing is very important. Typically, sperm lasts about 12 hours in the uterus; therefore, it is critical to get the sperm into the uterus as close as possible to egg release. The first appointment is an ultrasound 3-5 days after a woman's period to ensure she is not pregnant and that all reproductive parts look normal. At this appointment, women may opt to get a prescription for fertility medication, such as Letrozole or Chlomid, which are intended to increase follicle count. This means that rather than having one egg per cycle, the woman may release multiple eggs to improve the chances of fertilization. (Due to the higher chance of releasing and therefore fertilizing more than one egg, couples should deeply consider this prior to choosing this option.)

Note: Fertility drugs can play havoc with your hormones and emotional responses (they sure did with mine)! Prepare your wife, partner, co-workers, etc. for some heavy seas... and take your daily dose in the evening to avoid the biggest spikes in emotional irrationality. Also, even if your insurance doesn't cover the insemination appointments, there is a chance they will cover the fertility medication, so don't forget to check!

The next appointment is usually 7-10 days later. The doctor will count candidate follicles and measure to see if any are about to release an egg that has the potential to be fertilized. They will also check to make sure TOO many follicles aren't about to release eggs. Contrary to media sensations, fertility doctors see it as a failure if you end up with triplets+.

There are two options following this appointment: track ovulation via a test kit or receive a shot to force the release of an egg (ovulation). This is important as it allows women to know when ovulation will occur. The ovulation test kit is measuring your luteinizing hormone (LH) surge. Ovulation generally occurs 36 hours after this surge. The shot forces this surge to occur. Once you get a positive on the test kit or have the shot, call the fertility center immediately and schedule the insemination.

In addition to contacting the doctor to make an appointment, women need to understand the cryobank process as well. If the sperm is stored locally, the best option is to call the bank 4-7 days prior to ovulation to ensure the sperm and storage tank is available at the time of the appointment. If the sperm is not stored locally, it is recommended to have several vials shipped at a time for local storage because shipping can cost more than $200 dollars each time.

Reasons for Choosing IUI: IUI is a good choice for women who want to improve their chances of pregnancy, are willing to spend a little more, or have tried multiple ICIs without success. Because IUI is performed at the doctor's office, many lesbians I've spoken to (including myself) will skip ICI and go straight to IUI to (hopefully!) reduce the number of attempts necessary to be successful. Additionally, IUI is used for women that have cervical issues that do not allow sperm to enter into the uterus, or who do not have a regular cycle or release eggs properly. The chance of fertilization is up to 20 percent if the woman does not have any reproductive issues.

Real Stories: IUI

After 4 at-home ICI attempts, we decided to take stronger measures towards getting pregnant and went to a great fertility center near where we live. Our chosen donor only had IUI vials available so we decided to skip doctor-supported ICI and go straight to IUI. With ultrasounds and a lot of questions for the doctor, we learned a great deal more about my cycle. However, even with IUI and fertility medicine, it took us another 4 tries until we were finally successful. – Kathy and Lauren

We did un-medicated IUIs. Easiest, cheapest and the only route our doctor would start with because I was young-ish, ovulating, and healthy. – Tara and Tanya

In Vitro Fertilization (IVF)

IVF is the mack daddy of fertility treatments, taking fertilization out of the body and just leaving implantation up to us. But you'll be amazed at how many people think IVF is the only type of fertility treatment! I can't even tell you how many people asked us if we were doing IVF.

Description: The third, and most costly, option is IVF, In Vitro Fertilization. For IVF, the eggs are fertilized outside of the body in a lab and then placed back into the uterus for implantation. For lesbians, an added bonus to IVF is that one partner's eggs can be collected and then implanted into the other partner.

Basic Process: If you're considering the IVF route, it can be complicated and daunting. Insurance companies rarely cover the procedure. And your first appointment will usually cost around $250... Each. I'll walk through a lot of what they go over in the first consultation here. If you're serious about doing IVF down the road, it doesn't hurt to do the egg extraction early. Younger eggs are always better. Harvesting eggs a couple years early will lead to a minimal (compared to the overall expense of IVF) yearly storage fee, but the dividends from using younger eggs pay out in reduced risks of a host of genetic and chromosomal abnormalities the doctors will go over with you.

One big advantage lesbians have in this process (from my point of view) – usually we aren't going in because we haven't been able to get pregnant, but rather, we want to carry our wife's biological descendant. This means the level of stress we start with is much lower than couple that have struggled for years. And, as our doctor highlighted, keeping stress low is very important to getting pregnant.

The beginning stages of IVF are similar to IUI appointments. There are several appointments in which ultrasounds are performed, medications are administered, and the ovaries are stimulated into producing multiple mature eggs rather than one egg per cycle. When you're ready to schedule your first consultation, the clinic you choose will be very helpful about getting everything set up at the right times in your cycle and ordering labs you need to do before you arrive.

Before you even go to the appointment, you will both fill out a lot of paperwork and get blood work done. Then, when you arrive, the doctor will have a good picture of what your risk factors are. The first consultation will be scheduled separately, but some doctors will allow you to do them at the same time when you arrive. Either way, your spouse/partner can be present at the appointment. Following the consultation portion, the doctor will perform an intervaginal sonogram on both of you.

For the egg donor partner, the ultrasound will focus on the ovaries. The doctor will count the number of follicles you have on each ovary. Normal range is 5-20 follicles per ovary.

For the partner that will have the eggs transferred into her uterus, the focus of the scan will be the uterus itself. The doctor is checking for fibroids and other abnormalities and thickness of the lining wall.

Some states have additional things that will have to be checked, including the carrying mom's fallopian tubes via an HSG and that all the proper health checks were done on the donor sperm. If you got sperm from an unknown donor at a Cryobank, this was almost definitely done already. But if you are using a known donor there may be more things for you to verify.

Once everything is checked out, the doctor will be there to answer any additional questions you have before sending you to learn about the overall process from an administrative assistant and then finally, the financial advisor that lays out all the costs.

At the IVF facility we used, the egg harvest and transfer were priced at just under $13,000 and the cost of medications for the egg harvest were projected to be between $4 and $8k. They can't predict all the costs because they won't know until the medicine is administered how an individual will respond.

The egg harvest partner can expect to go through a couple weeks of birth control and then a period of 10-14 days where they are on heavy estrogen to get many eggs to ripen. During this time, there will be almost daily checkups and ultrasounds. All of these will be well coordinated by your clinic. When they are ready to harvest, the egg harvestee will be put under anesthetic and an ultrasound will be used to guide a needle that will suck the sonovial fluid (and the eggs) from your follicles. The procedure lasts about 15 min.

The egg is then fertilized in a lab using the donor sperm. This is the major difference between ICI or IUI and IVF treatments: the fertilization does not happen naturally in the woman's body, but rather outside. The fertilized eggs will be monitored for a few days to ensure they are developing properly, and then it will be transferred back into the uterus. For women with no history of reproductive issues, one embryo may be transferred in order to avoid the risk of having multiple embryos stick; however, for women with a history of failed IVF treatments, doctors may suggest using more than one embryo. This stage is very quick and does not require any sedation, and both partners can be present to watch it happen on a screen.

Throughout the entire 10-14 days and then 2-4 days after the harvest, the patient is required to be very careful and avoid high impact activities. There are risks to walking around with more mature eggs than your body would normally produce, such as Ovarian

Hyperstimulation Syndrome, which is rare condition that typically occurs in less than 5% of harvestees. Severe cases of this syndrome may result in damage to the ovaries. In less severe cases, they may experience severe bloating and strong cramping. If you show symptoms consistent with hyperstimulation, your physician may reduce your medication dosage or terminate the egg donation cycle to avoid medical complications.

Once the eggs are extracted, the fertility center makes all the magic happen, combining the eggs and sperm, allowing them to gestate to the 5-day mark to see which ones are viable, performing any testing you request, and then freezing them until you are ready to implant them into the carrying mom's uterus.

When you decide you are ready to attempt an implantation, you will track your cycle and be put on certain medicines to help prepare your uterus and encourage implantation.

Reasons for Choosing IVF: Because of the expense, IVF was intended and is recommended for partners who have not had success with other attempts at fertilization, are over 40, or fear any genetic problems. However, this procedure may also be the right choice for lesbian couples in which one mother wishes to donate the egg while the other mother wishes to carry the baby to term.

Real Stories: IVF

We chose IVF based on our age and the percentage of success being slightly higher. We also did not have a plethora of donor sperm and it was the only option we could use if I was going to carry Lisa's egg. – Kayla and Lisa

In our family, I am the one that wants to carry and my wife is completely ok without doing so. However, for our second child, I know I want her genetic offspring so we will be doing IVF – harvesting her eggs and implanting the embryo in my uterus. – Kathy and Lauren

IVF was our last resort due to cost and lack of intimacy in the process. – Asha and Marissa

Making the decision to have a baby can be difficult and exciting enough without having to worry about how it is going to happen. Hopefully this break down of the three different procedures that allow you to carry your own child and use your own genes helps clear up some of the confusion. The decision between whether to use ICI, IUI, or IVF is ultimately up to you and must take into consideration who will carry the baby, who will donate the egg, who will donate the sperm, the allowed budget, and the reproductive health of all parties involved. Also, if you do IVF, you'll also have to decide what to do with any leftover embryos.

Chapter 8 Assignment: Figure out which method is best for you to start with based on the research you did into your insurance carrier, local fertility centers, and cryobanks.

Chapter 9. Costs of Making a Family and How to Avoid the Costs You Can

There are many costs involved with artificial insemination, including some obvious ones like doctor visits and some less obvious ones like ovulation test kits. Different insurance plans vary wildly, covering none, some, or all types of fertility treatments (though I haven't found any that will pay for sperm). Even insurance plans that won't cover the artificial insemination may still cover some of the medicines required. The key is to always ask. And if you speak to someone that doesn't sound very sure, ask to speak to another representative that knows more.

Costs that Affect All Types of Artificial Insemination

Item	Cost	How to Save $
Blood Work	$0-$200	This is often covered by insurance so don't forget to check. Also, you may have already had some of the tests done recently enough, so double check.
Ovulation Test	From $20 for 20	Use the cheapest

Item	Cost	How to Save $
Kits	strips to $20 per digital test stick	method (test strips)
Pregnancy Tests	$12-$20 for a pack of 3	Look online for bulk discounts
Cryobank Membership and Additional Donor Information	$30 per piece of information to $250 for 3 months of access	Research which one is the best option for you before committing to a subscription plan
Cryobank Storage	$0 - $1000+/year	See what deals you can get when you purchase sperm or what discounts they have
Sperm shipping	$180-$300/shipment	Determine if it would be more cost effective to pay for storage at a local cryobank so you only have to pay for shipping once.
Sperm, Known donor, fresh	$0 to any price you negotiated	
Sperm, Known donor, donated through a cryobank (Directed Donor)	$200-$1000 for consultation, genetic testing, and physical	

Item	Cost	How to Save $
Sperm, Unknown donor, ICI vials (washed once)	Sperm: $500-$800	Some spermbanks will give you a discount if you order above a certain number of vials
Sperm, Unknown donor, IUI vials (washed twice)	$600-$900	Some spermbanks will give you a discount if you order above a certain number of vials

The Cost of ICI (IntraCervical Insemination)

The cost of ICI can vary depending on the type of sperm donated and who it came from. If the procedure is done at home with a known sperm donor at no cost, the procedure can cost under $100 per attempt. When done at a clinic, the price can range from $100 - $600, though the price goes up if sperm is washed or frozen during the visit, plus the cost of the sperm.

Item	Cost
ICI Procedures - At home	$3 (needleless syringes)
ICI Procedures - At the doctor's office – no ultrasound	$100-$300
ICI Procedures - At the doctor's office – ultrasound	$100-$600

Note: Many cryobanks will buy back unused vials.

The Cost of IUI (IntraUterine Insemination)

Item	Cost
IUI Procedure - Initial Consultation	$100-$500
IUI Procedure - Ultrasound Visits	$100-$300
IUI Procedure - Insemination Visit	$100-$300
IUI Procedure - Fertility Drugs	$5 co-pay - $100
IUI Procedure - Sperm Preparation	$100-$300

The Cost of IVF (In Vitro Fertilization)

IVF treatments are significantly more costly than the other two options. An average cycle can cost from $12,000-$20,000. Clinics can vary greatly for their cost, so it is best to research your local ones. Additionally, some clinics offer different types of financing – from payment plans to buy 7 attempts up front and get your money back if none are successful (though this last one is typically only recommended for people that are having big problems getting pregnant).

Chapter 9 Assignment: Sit down with the budget you reviewed in Chapter 1 and figure out which artificial insemination methods fit within your budget. If none of them do, discuss ways to put money away. Be prepared to have to escalate to more expensive methods if the first ones don't work initially.

Real Stories: Did your insurance cover any part of the process?

No. We were grateful that our savings covered all expenses for the [IVF] procedure. We did not have to commit to monthly payments or debt. – Kayla and Lisa

Our insurance carrier didn't cover any infertility treatments. Luckily, I am a veteran of the US Navy and at one of my VA check-ups I mentioned to my doctor that we were trying to have a baby. I was very pleasantly surprised to discover that the VA actually covers certain types of fertility treatment under their Women's Health program. We were referred out to an amazing fertility center for IUI (which will be described later) at no cost to us. – Kathy and Lauren

The fertility clinic treats you like a straight person experiencing fertility issues. My insurance covered all the diagnostic testing. – Tara and Tanya

Our insurance would cover $10k, but for us it was way cheaper to pay a personal donor. – Asha and Marissa

Chapter 10. What to Expect at Your First Doctor Visit

At your first appointment, you should expect a vaginal ultrasound. This should not be painful, but about or slightly less uncomfortable as a PAP smear. A small probe is inserted into the vagina to get a good picture of the uterus in order to make sure you aren't pregnant, and to check out the uterus, ovaries, and fallopian tubes.

The doctor will also check your follicle count. Follicles are the sacks that store the eggs until they are mature. The follicle grows with the egg, and prior to ovulation, the follicle with the best candidate will release its egg from the ovary. Another thing that will be checked out is your cervix. This is the narrower, bottom portion of the uterus. The cervix helps weed out sperm that are weak or dead to make sure the strongest candidates survive, and also releases cervical mucus. Cervical mucus is at its highest quality after surging an egg, and it assists and nourishes sperm on their way to the egg. How well the cervix looks and the quality of the mucus can determine which type of insemination to choose.

After insemination, the fun part begins: checking for pregnancy. But first, doctors must check out the uterus to make sure there is nothing wrong, because the uterus is where the baby grows. The health of the uterus is important because it needs a thick lining for the egg to be implanted and nourished. After conception, the fertilized egg released a hormone known as HCG.

Elevated presence of this hormone in urine or blood indicates if you are pregnant.

Now, let the testing begin! There are two key types of pregnancy tests: home pregnancy tests are the typical "pee on a stick" device that checks for the HCG hormone in urine. These tests are very cheap, ranging from $5-20 depending on the brand. The other type is a blood test in a doctor's office which checks for HCG in the blood. The cost varies from $25-100. It is more expensive because blood is drawn, but it can show results sooner than home pregnancy tests.

Chapter 10 Assignment: When you're ready, make your first doctor's appointment!

Real Stories: Choosing a doctor/fertility center

Research the facilities that provide IVF/IUI procedures and consider their success rates, history and reviews. For example, the reviews of the doctor we chose said he was not good with bed-side manner - which actually worked better for me. The touchy-feely type wasn't the doctor for me. I wanted to go in, get the tests, go through the procedure and have it be more like a business transaction. Other women I know prefer to feel more warmth or kindness or laughs or rapport. So analyze your needs in that area too. – Kayla and Lisa

Chapter 11. Fertility Drugs and Their Effects on You (Brace Yourself for Crazy)

I'm not going to go into detail here about all the different types of fertility drugs and their scientific effects – your doctor will definitely do all of that with you. I just want to go over quickly how they might make you feel.

Now, not everyone is going to need them and not every doctor is going to recommend you take them until other options have been tried and exhausted. But for those of you that do end up being prescribed them, there are things to be aware of.

Fertility drugs directly affect the level of hormones in your body. And if you think back to a time when you knew your period was coming because you felt bloated and crabby, that will give you a small glimpse into what fertility drugs may be like for you. Some drugs will affect you more than others and the doctor can modify the dosage he prescribes you.

As an example, for me, chlomid made me extremely, irrationally angry. I was not the most pleasant person to be around. I told my doctor about this and on the next cycle he switched me to letrozole and recommended I take it at night so that the bulk of my craziness would occur while I slept. That made a huge difference for me (and those around me!).

I don't share this so you will shy away from fertility drugs, only so that you know there are many side effects and they can each affect you differently. Talk to your doctor about all the side effects so you can be ready. Talk to any friends you have that went through something like this so you can learn about effective ways to handle your mood swings.

And, if all these fertility drugs are successful, just remember that pregnancy is its own special hormone cocktail so you and your partner are in for quite a ride!

Real Stories: The Varying Effects of Chlomid

Interestingly, I found out that because I was on chlomid, my cycle stretched from 22 – 25 days to 28 – 30 days. So every time I thought I was pregnant around day 26, I took a test, it was negative, and then I got my period a couple days later. Once I learned about the delay due to chlomid, I was able to chill out and wait until day 31 to take a pregnancy test. – Kathy and Lauren

Chapter 12. Awkward Questions Strangers Will Ask

Strangers ask the most intimate questions. Over the last two years (a year of trying + pregnancy), we've been asked A LOT of awkward questions about our decisions and processes for getting pregnant. Now, I don't think people intentionally ask these questions to be awkward or weird, they just don't realize how PERSONAL some of these questions really are. When lesbians ask them, I usually get the feeling like they want to know so that they have other viewpoints to consider in their own decision making process. When straight people ask them, I sometimes feel like a zoo creature getting a colonoscopy in front of a packed crowd.

The most important thing about all these questions is that, as a couple, you've considered them and are on the same page with your answers. Even the most open, tell-all partners can suddenly clam up and not want to share every detail of your pregnancy journey. Take the time to decide together what you as a couple are comfortable to share with others.

Who is the dad?
This one always bugs me for a couple reasons. First, our donor is in no way a "dad" or even "father." Like countless other non-traditional families (single parents, steps, blended, adopted, etc.) genetic ties do not dictate parental rights. Second, when's the last time you went

up to a straight couple that obviously had adopted children and asked them who the parents are? And finally, I've never gone up to a straight couple in the waiting room at the fertility clinic and asked, "Hey, so if he can't produce the goods, who's going to be the dad?" The truth is, the genetics of our baby are irrelevant to anyone except my wife and I.

Who is the mom?

People are curious about who carried the baby because they think it matters which genes the baby carries. But it doesn't. We stopped answering this question when our son was born.

Are you going known or unknown donor?

It took us months of soul searching, tons of research, and many vulnerable conversations to decide on this one. No, I'm not going to tell you, person-that-I-just-met, because you're curious. The only other parent this baby will ever have is my wife. My wife and I have a canned response for this one that makes a little joke of it while giving away no details.

Must be nice to get to pick the genes your baby will get. My husband isn't exactly Brad Pitt.

I know women that say this are trying to be funny and/or look on the bright side, but this question kills me on the inside a little bit every time it is asked. I would do ANYTHING to have a baby that was a genetic combination of my wife and me. But science isn't quite there so I generally make a joke about picking a genius, pro-sport playing Adonis and then move on quickly.

How are you going to do it?

This one seems innocent the first time you hear it but if you think about it a little more, you realize they asked you a question about your vagina. In reality, we didn't have any issues with this question. A lot of women asked it, and surprisingly, many of them followed up with their own tails of infertility issues and procedures. It turns out society has a bit of a taboo around talking about fertility issues. When straight women in this situation find out a lesbian couple is inseminating, they immediately know that it's not a standard birds-and-bees operation. We really learned a lot from the women that asked us this question.

How did you decide who would carry? Did you flip a coin?

Um, yes, we flipped a coin because that's how we make all of our major life decisions.

Are you going to make your wife carry next time?

This one makes me laugh because I have yet to "make" my wife do anything. We generally prefer to sit down and have rational conversations where we both lay out our preferences and take into consideration the many choices available to us and then come to a mutually agreed upon decision. Because we are grown ups. In a grown up relationship.

Are your parents ok with it?

There are a lot of ways to ask this question. This particular way makes me want to throat punch the person asking. I understand that they are curious to see if my baby's grandparents will be supportive. But when asked if someone is "ok" with something, it implies their consent is necessary for us to have this baby. And I can't remember the last time I heard someone ask a straight couple if their parents were ok with it... unless that couple was in high school. The only people my wife and I give our real answer to for this question are very close friends that already know our situation with our respective parents.

Are you worried they will be teased/ostracized for having two mommies?

If only this was my only worry for our future child(ren). There are so many reasons kids get teased (hair color, weight, first name rhymes with..., clothing choices, etc.) that having two moms (especially since we live in California) is probably the least of their concerns. We have to hope that the love we give them will be more than enough.

Prepare Yourselves in Advance

Some of these questions are funny, many could be awkward, and there's a lot of personal stuff behind each answer. Any time a new question was asked of my wife or me, we'd answer it a little awkwardly and then talk about it later. We both wanted to make sure that we were ok with sharing the information. With a new baby looming on the horizon, we like the idea of practicing our teamwork before we're pressured by a two year old determined to get his/her own way!

Chapter 12 Assignment: Go through all these awkward questions with each other to get on the same page about how you answer them.

Real Stories: Talking about the uncomfortable stuff

Talk about the known expectations and acknowledge the possible disappointments that might occur. Talk about all the uncomfortable stuff. Ideas of donors, what's important what's not. For me, I always thought that if it wasn't "my" baby that I wouldn't feel as connected or "part" of the journey. Wow, was I wrong (I guess it's a bit different since I carried Lisa's baby - but it was definitely a concern of mine). I have heard this concern from other women I know that are considering their own journeys, but talk about that stuff. – Kayla and Lisa

Chapter 13. Taking Care of You and Staying Sane During the Process

Start Taking Care of Your Body Now

The road to becoming pregnant is filled with many ups and downs. This can be a time of great anxiety, but also a time of anticipation and excitement. This emotional roller coaster can be highly stressful on any couple attempting to conceive, no matter how long they have been trying or how many other kids they may have. This preconception period is an important time, however. Most doctors agree that the physical and emotional health of the mother at this juncture can and will affect her pregnancy and the health of her baby-to-be. Here are some major points that lesbian couples trying to conceive need to be aware of surrounding the preconception period.

Diet

When trying to conceive, what you eat and any supplements you take can potentially affect your pregnancy. A well-balanced diet with the appropriate calorie content for the woman's dietary needs is important, as it will affect her upcoming pregnancy. Pre-natal vitamins should also be taken from about three months prior to the desired time of conception. Most doctors will recommend taking folic acid also, as most women don't get enough of it and a deficiency has been proven to directly affect the fetus. During pregnancy, the body needs sufficient stores of iron, vitamin C and D, fiber calcium, and folic acid.

Folic acid, also known as folate, is extremely important in pregnancy. It is a type of B vitamin that promotes normal nerve functioning and helps in the production of red blood cells. Women who have low levels of folate have been proven to have an increased risk of having a baby with spinal cord and brain abnormalities, such as spina bifida. If a woman has no history of a neural tube defect, she should aim for 400 micrograms per day. Good sources of folic acid include beans, green vegetables such as spinach and broccoli, oranges, raspberries, cantaloupe, and enriched breads and cereals.

Body Weight

Women trying to conceive should also aim to have a healthy body weight prior to conception. Obesity will increase the risk for several issues in pregnancy, such as miscarriage, diabetes, preeclampsia, and neural tube defects. Being overweight or underweight can also increase infertility in women. Women trying to conceive should get adequate amounts of sleep, which will help maintain a healthy weight. Sleeping 7-8 hours each night is ideal, and less than 6 can be unhealthy. Women should aim to exercise at least three times per week. In addition, reducing emotional stress can help decrease emotional eating.

Harmful Exposures

Women trying to conceive should make every attempt to stop smoking prior to conceiving. Smoking can decrease fertility and increase the risk of miscarriage, pre-term delivery, and low birth weight. In fact, second-hand smoke, or passive smoke, can increase these risk almost as much as first-hand smoke. If the partner who will not be getting pregnant does smoke, she should do so outdoors, away from the other partner, or attempt to quit altogether. There has never been a better reason to do so.

Caffeine should be limited to 200mg, or 1-2 cups, per day. Too much caffeine can potentially increase the risks of miscarriage and preterm birth. Mothers to be and their partners should understand that caffeine is found in more than just coffee, but also in chocolate, tea, energy drinks, most sodas, and aspirin products.

Alcohol and recreational drugs should also be avoided by women attempting to conceive. At the point, a lesbian couple decides to start a fertility journey, the partner who will carry their baby should act as if she were pregnant. This means she would not want to expose her unborn baby to various alcohol and recreational drugs, so she should not do it prior to conception either. Alcohol and many drugs taken during pregnancy can lead to mental retardation, stunted growth, low birth weight, stillbirth, severe birth defects, and even newborn addiction to the substance at delivery. Taking alcohol and recreational drugs prior to conceiving or during a pregnancy is simply not worth the risk for the mom or the baby.

Prescription, Over the Counter, and Herbal Medications

All other medications a potential mother-to-be needs or wants to take should be discussed with their OB/GYN. Some drugs can be taken safely during this time period and during pregnancy, and others cannot. It is best to play it safe and check with a physician first.

Other Exposures

During preconception and pregnancy, women should stay away from lead paint. This is especially true if they live in an older home, where many older paints were made with lead. Home repairs like sanding and scraping can send lead dust into the air, potentially causing problems for the mother and unborn baby.

Women hoping to conceive soon should also stay away from radiation, most commonly in the form of x-rays. If they require an x-ray, they should let the radiology tech know that they are attempting to be or possibly pregnant at that time.

Reducing Stress

During the preconception period, both partners should focus on reducing stress. Women who are under a lot of stress, particularly in regards to conceiving, can actually reduce their chances of getting pregnant. Taking some time to focus on parts of life that have nothing to do with babies or conceiving can be a good stress relief for lesbian couples at this time. Focusing on each other, as well as hobbies, pets, traveling, cooking, crafting, and on the relationship itself can all be good forms of stress relief to give the mind and body a break from the journey to conceive.

A source of stress most people don't think about is the two weeks after insemination that you think and act like you might be pregnant, only to be followed by a huge let down if you weren't successful. After a couple of failed attempts, the stress can increase greatly. Recognize that this may be an issue and find ways to de-stress. This may even mean taking a month or two break just to climb off the emotional roller coaster!

Real Stories: How long did it take you to get pregnant?

Twice. Each IVF transfer consisted of two fertilized eggs. – Kayla and Lisa

Two months (we inseminated twice each month). – Tara and Tanya

One year with eight tries. We took a couple months off because we were worried the stress was contributing to our challenges. The next time we tried, we succeeded. – Kathy and Lauren

On and off over a year and a half. – Asha and Marissa

Above all, women should try to relax and enjoy this special time in their lives. Lesbian couples should speak to their doctors with further questions regarding the preconception period, tips on trying to conceive or having a healthy pregnancy.

Even with all the knowledge you now have of your body's inner workings from this book, you may still feel confused or lost, but there are many resources available on the Internet to attain more information on fertility, artificial insemination, conception, or pregnancy in general. The American Pregnancy Organization has an abundance of information on all of these topics. The BabyCenter website also has a wealth of information on fertility and pregnancy, as well forums and blogs to read about others experiences, or to get answers to some of your concerns while moving through the process. Ultimately, your doctor is the best resource you can have as they will be guiding you through this wonderful journey of starting a family.

Real Stories: How did you feel when you found out you were pregnant?

Surprised and elated. Blessed. – Asha and Marissa

The most excited I'd ever been about anything. When it was time to test the month I got pregnant, I woke up, peed on the stick and went back to bed to wait. Tanya got up and went to the bathroom and I told her to read the test. She looked at it (without her glasses on) and said it was negative. She left it on the counter and came back to bed. I cried and was upset but went back to sleep. An hour or so later when I woke up, I went back to the bathroom and picked up the test to throw it away. I examined it and noticed that it actually had two pink lines, I was pregnant!! I started laughing and screaming and ran back to show Tanya but I wasn't sure if I could was because the test had been sitting. I immediately

*took another and discovered I was indeed pregnant. —
Tara and Tanya*

*I cried immediately and called my mother. I called her
before Lisa I think! I wanted her arms around me. I was
frightened, happy, sad, in love and in shock all in the
same moment. I felt everything. – Kayla and Lisa*

*We'd tried so many times that I stopped taking
pregnancy tests until at least day 32 of my cycle
(pregnancy tests were expensive and had been
disappointing so many times!). We were so unconcerned
about taking the test that Lauren had taken a work trip
around testing time. I woke up on day 32 and thought,
what the heck, no period yet, I guess I'll pee on that
stick. When the 2 lines popped up, I couldn't believe it! I
took a picture and texted it to her. When she didn't call
me immediately, I called her. I was crying and excited
and she got really worried. It turned out she hadn't seen
the text yet! – Kathy and Lauren*

Thank you for reading this book. I really hope it helps!

ABOUT THE AUTHOR

Kathy Borkoski was a confused lesbian in 2013. She and her wife knew they wanted to get pregnant but couldn't figure it out easily. After googling, reading, researching, and hounding anyone they met that had gone through any kind of fertility treatments, they finally figured out just enough to get pregnant and start an adorable family. Of course, any lesbian that saw Kathy's gigantic belly knew that she probably had some insight into making that magic happen, so they asked her all their burning questions about how they could get pregnant, too.

And so the idea for a book that lays out how to help lesbians make a baby was born.

Kathy sincerely hopes that this book results in at least one adorable baby – namely, yours!

Find out more on: http://lesbianconception101.com

Follow us on Facebook:
www.facebook.com/TwoMomsPregnancyConception101

Follow us on Twitter: @Become2Moms

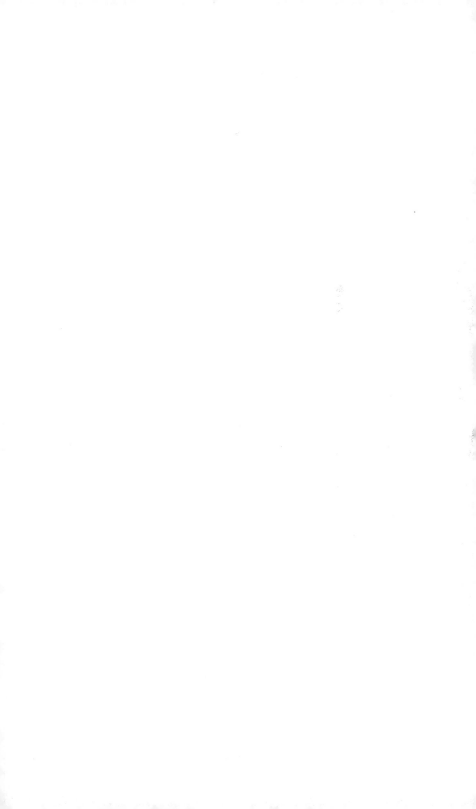

Printed in Great Britain
by Amazon